LU☾ID
HOUSE
PUBLISHING

Published in Marietta, Georgia, United States of America
by Lucid House Publishing, LLC LucidHousePublishing.com
©Copyright 2025 by Intact America
Photographs ©Copyright 2025 by Kevin N. Garrett
All rights reserved. First Edition.
Designer: Hector Sanchez
Production: The Design Lab Atlanta, Inc.
Editorial Coordinator: Echo Montgomery Garrett

Library of Congress Cataloging-in-Publication Data:
Intact America
Skin in the game: circumcision cuts through us all/by Intact America
and photography by Kevin N. Garrett—1st Edition
Print ISBN 978-1-950495-68-9

MED058090, FAM038000

GRIEF.
ANGER. SHOCK.
DISBELIEF.
SHAME. REGRET.
DEPRESSION.
RAGE.
REVULSION.
DYSFUNCTION.
DISSOCIATION.
TRAUMA.

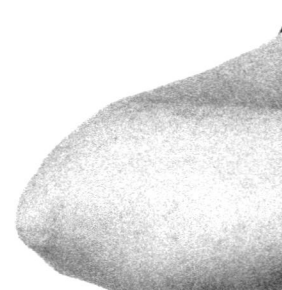

No matter what language you speak, these images communicate the range of emotions sparked by the routine cutting of the genitals of babies and children, who cannot consent yet are subjected to this irreversible, life-altering surgery. Since 2008, **Intact America** has been working to reveal the truth about the harm the most common pediatric surgery in the United States causes to baby boys, the men they become, and everyone in that person's intimate circle, who loves them.

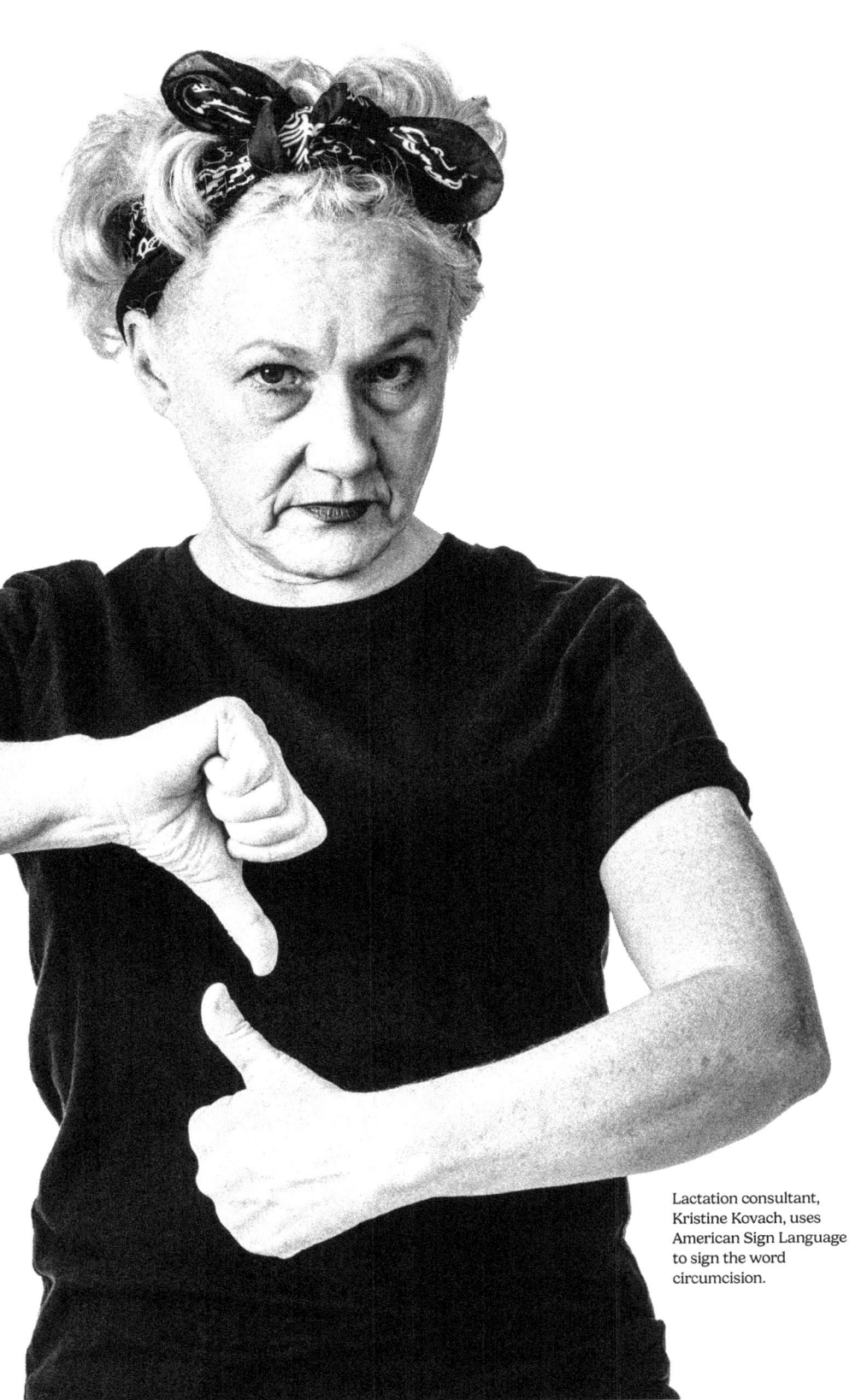

Lactation consultant, Kristine Kovach, uses American Sign Language to sign the word circumcision.

**USE YOUR VOICE.
ADVOCATE.
RECOGNIZE.
EMPATHIZE.
APOLOGIZE.
SPREAD THE WORD.
SAY NO TO
CIRCUMCISION.
HEAL BY REVEALING.**

Intact America gives people a safe place to share their stories. Knowing that you are not alone in your pain and feeling truly heard is often the first step to healing trauma.

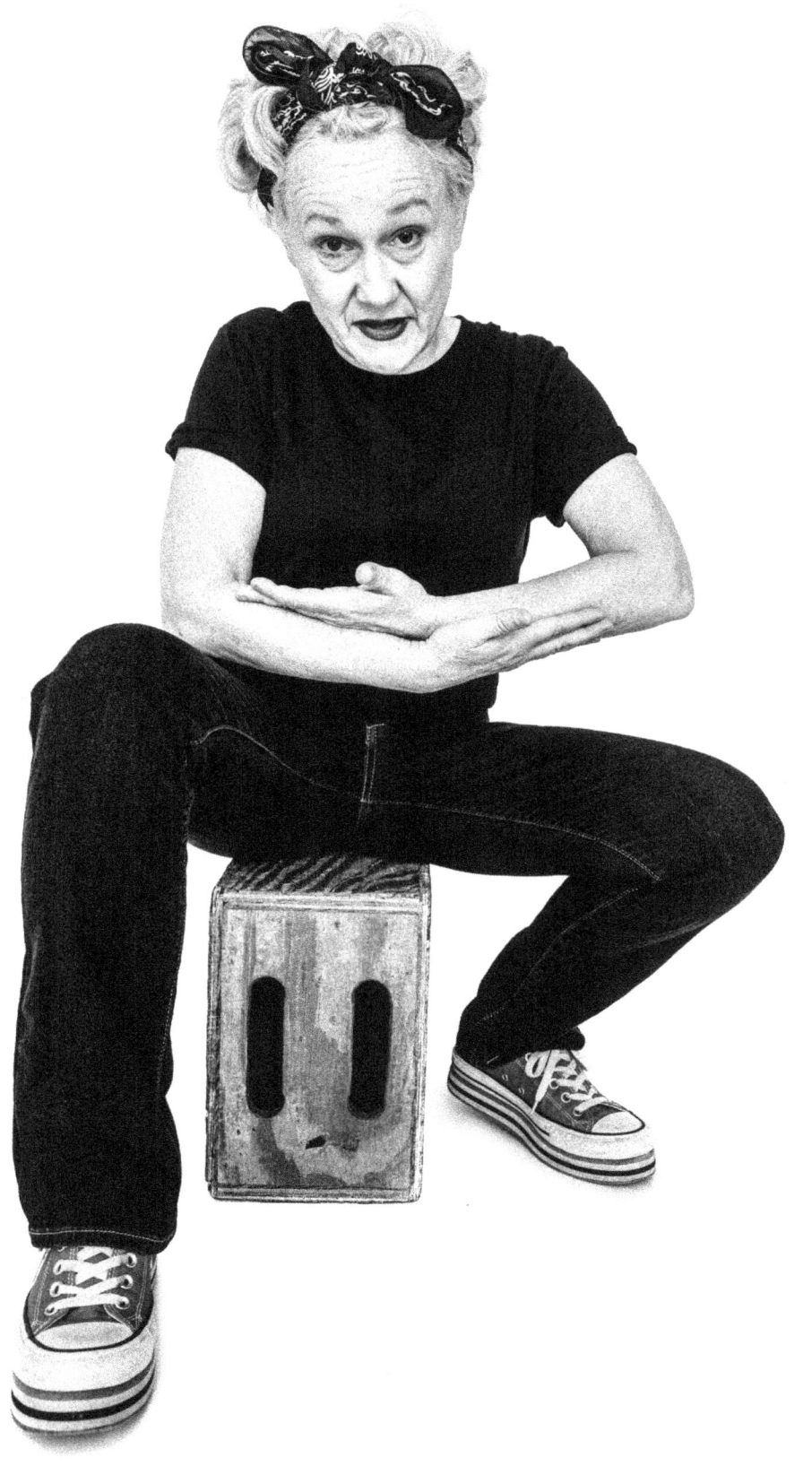

OUR STORIES CONNECT US.

When **Intact America (IA)** launched our *Voices* series in 2017, we had trouble finding even one person willing to reveal their name and send a photo to publish with the story of the damage they had suffered from having their genitals cut as helpless babies or children. Now more and more people have found the price of secrecy and self-repression too great to endure. This groundswell of people aching to tell their truths paved the way for **Intact America's** story-telling photo campaign, called **"SKIN IN THE GAME: Circumcision Cuts Through Us All,"** photographed by **Kevin Garrett** and designed by **Hector Sanchez**.

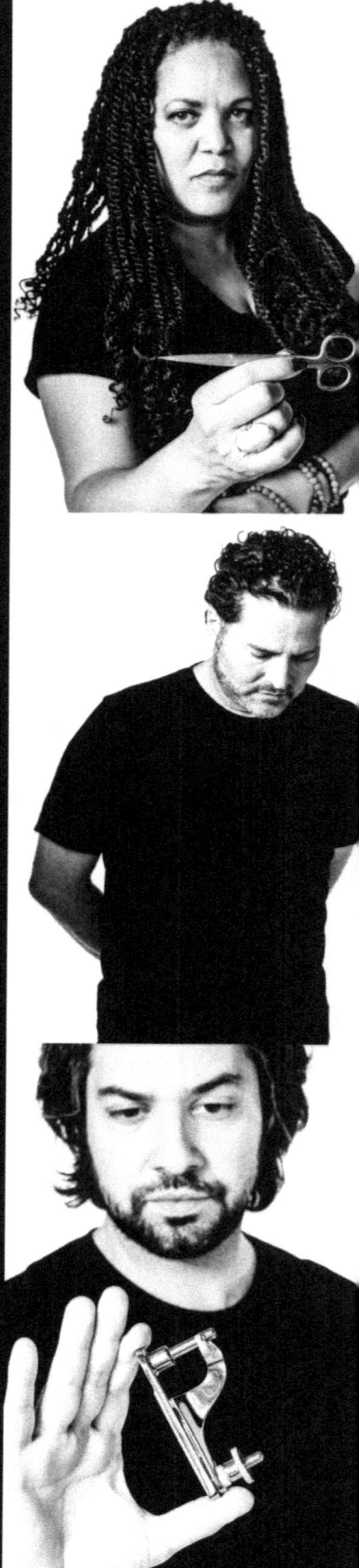

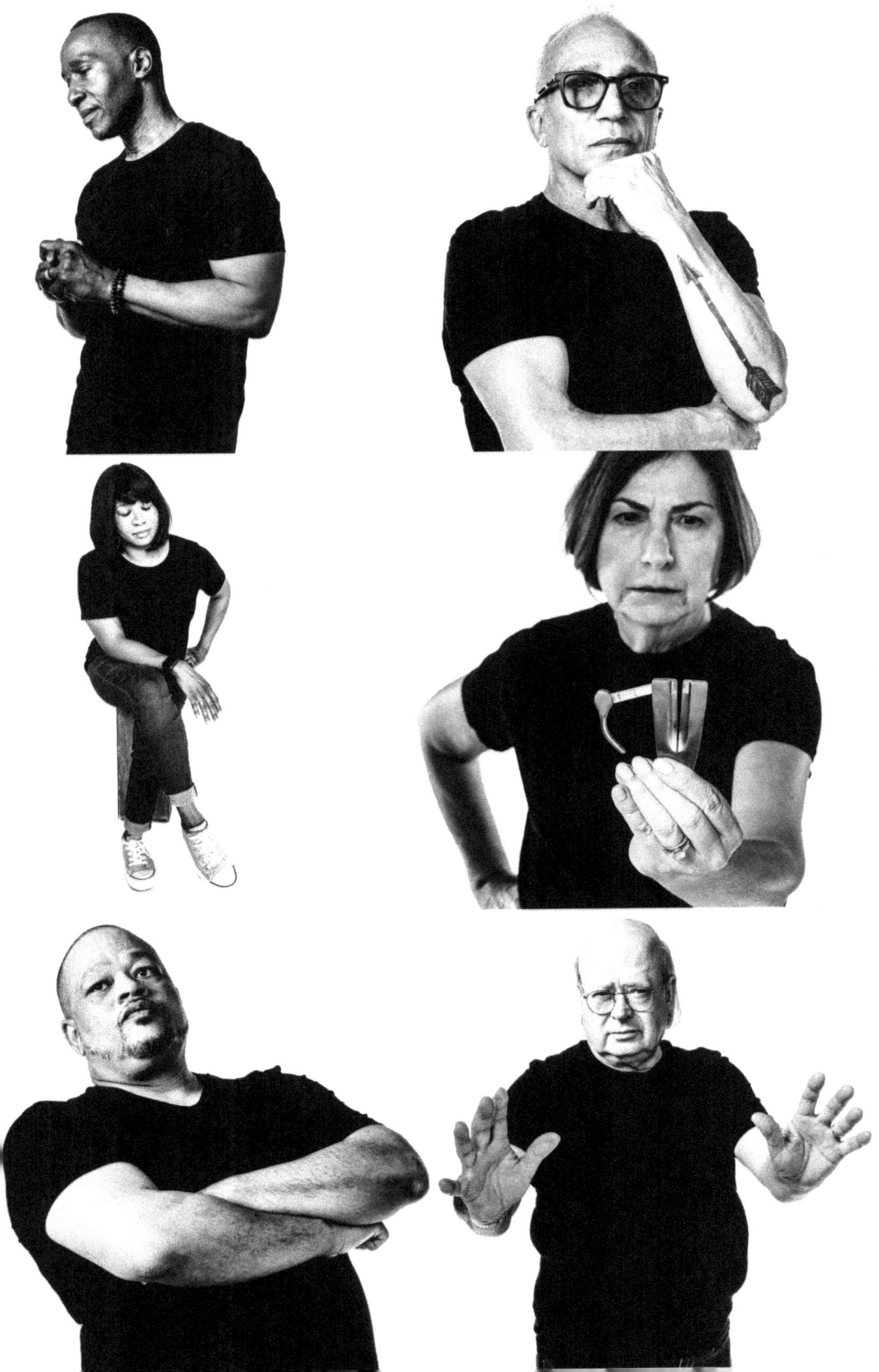

Doctors thought they could do *whatever* they wanted.

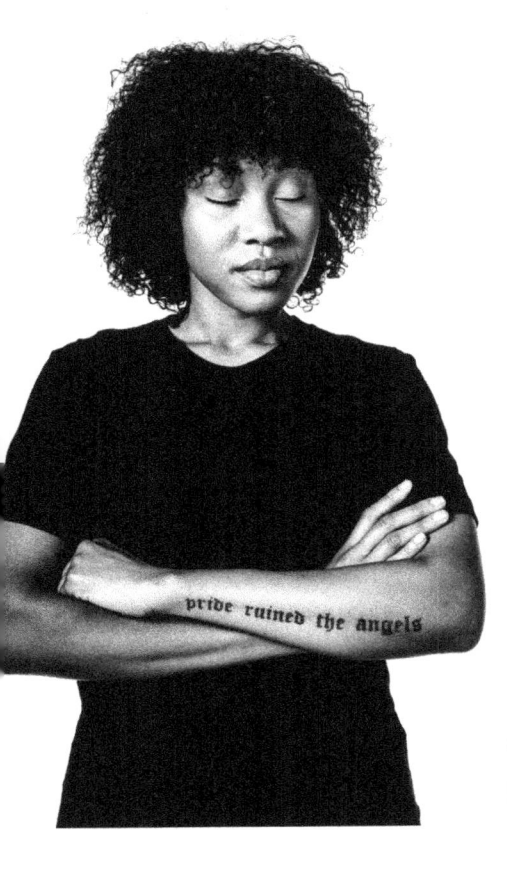
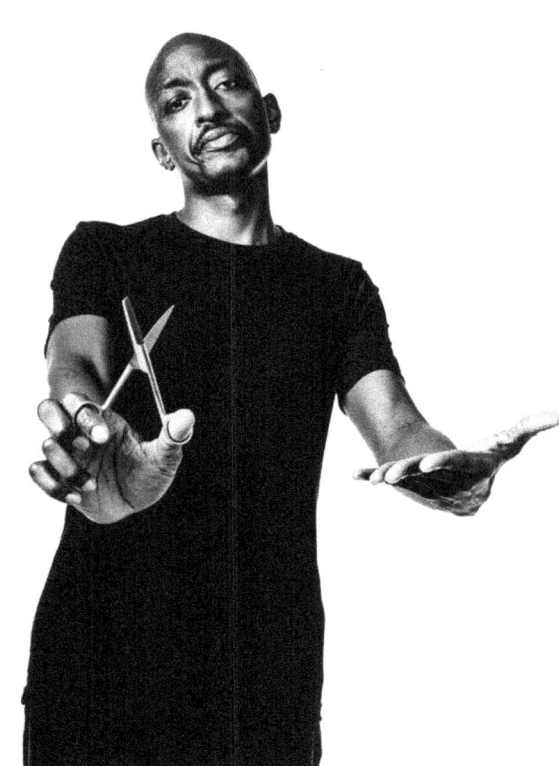
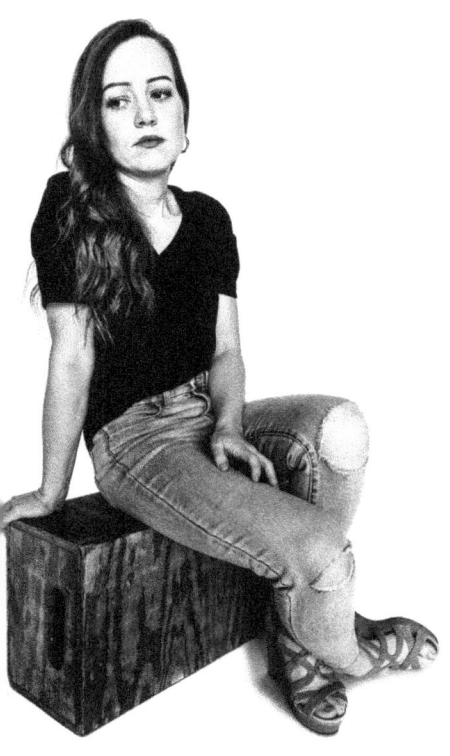
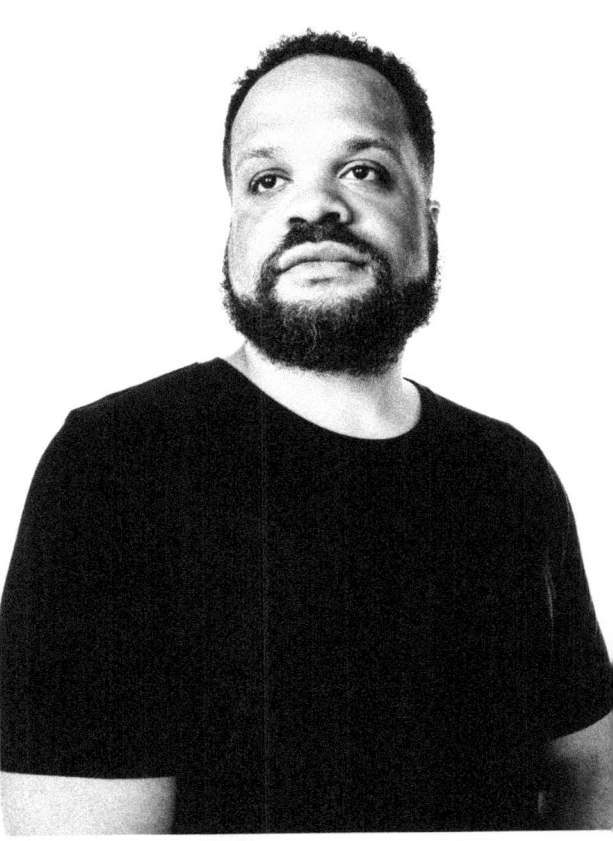

THE POWER OF LISTENING FROM THE HEART. THE MAGIC OF BEING HEARD.

The campaign photographs were taken in a series of three photo shoots, two in Atlanta and one in Dallas in 2023. Most participants were unknown to IA before they responded to online ads inviting interested people of any race, ethnicity, sex, and body type to have their pictures taken and share their circumcision story. Some said they'd been thinking about the harms of circumcision for years; others said they had never consciously considered the harm until they saw the ad. We met people of all ages, of every sexual orientation. The atmosphere was magical. As the hours and days progressed, we realized that virtually everyone in our country has a circumcision story to share whether they know it or not. The resulting photos and quotes of participants are intensely emotional. They affirm the vital ongoing work of Intact America and illustrate the important messages of the two memoirs by leaders in the intactivist movement, **This Penis Business** by **Georganne Chapin** with Echo Montgomery Garrett and **Please Don't Cut the Baby!** by **Marilyn Fayre Milos** with Judy Kirkwood {2024, Lucid House Publishing}.

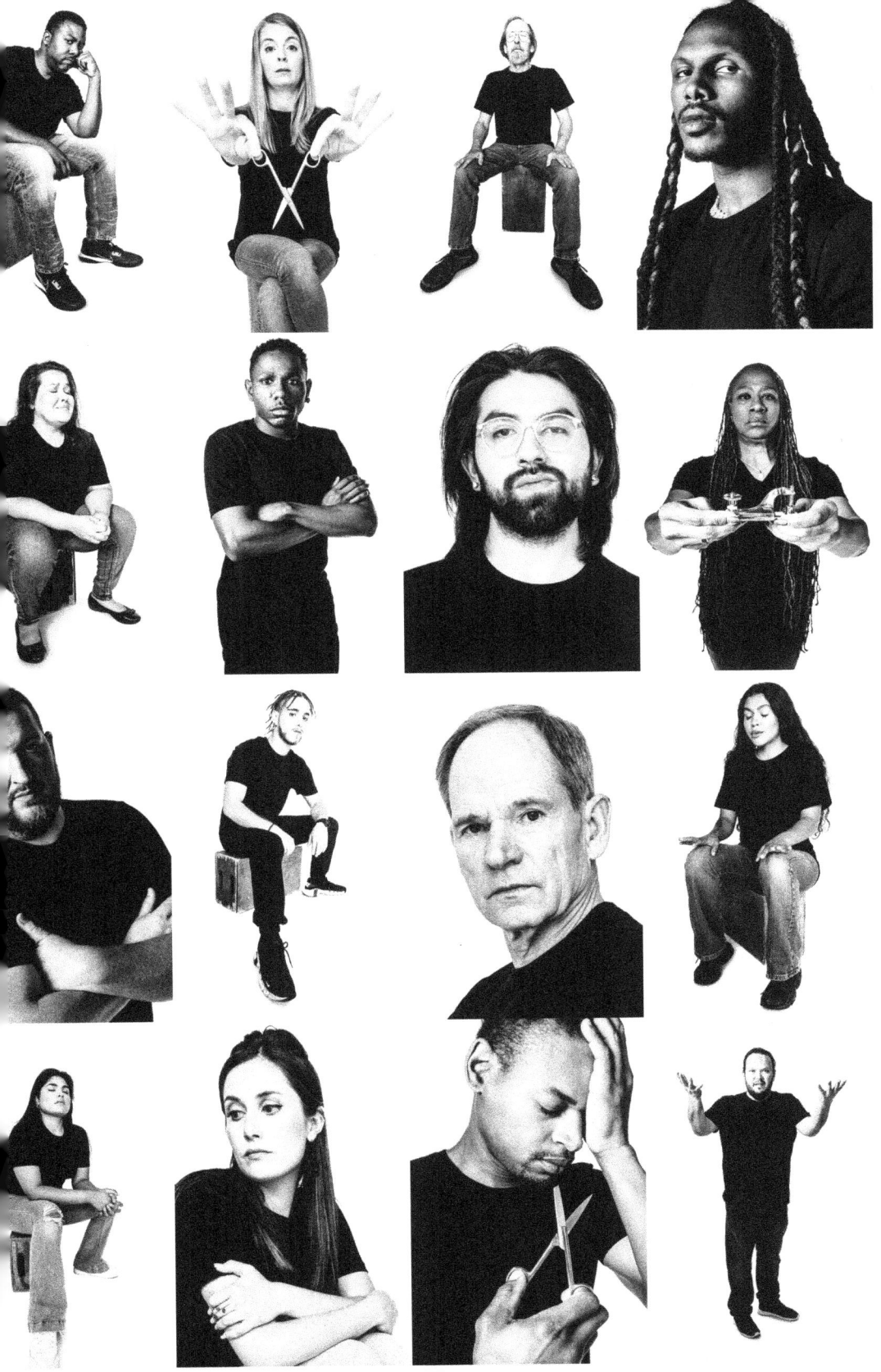

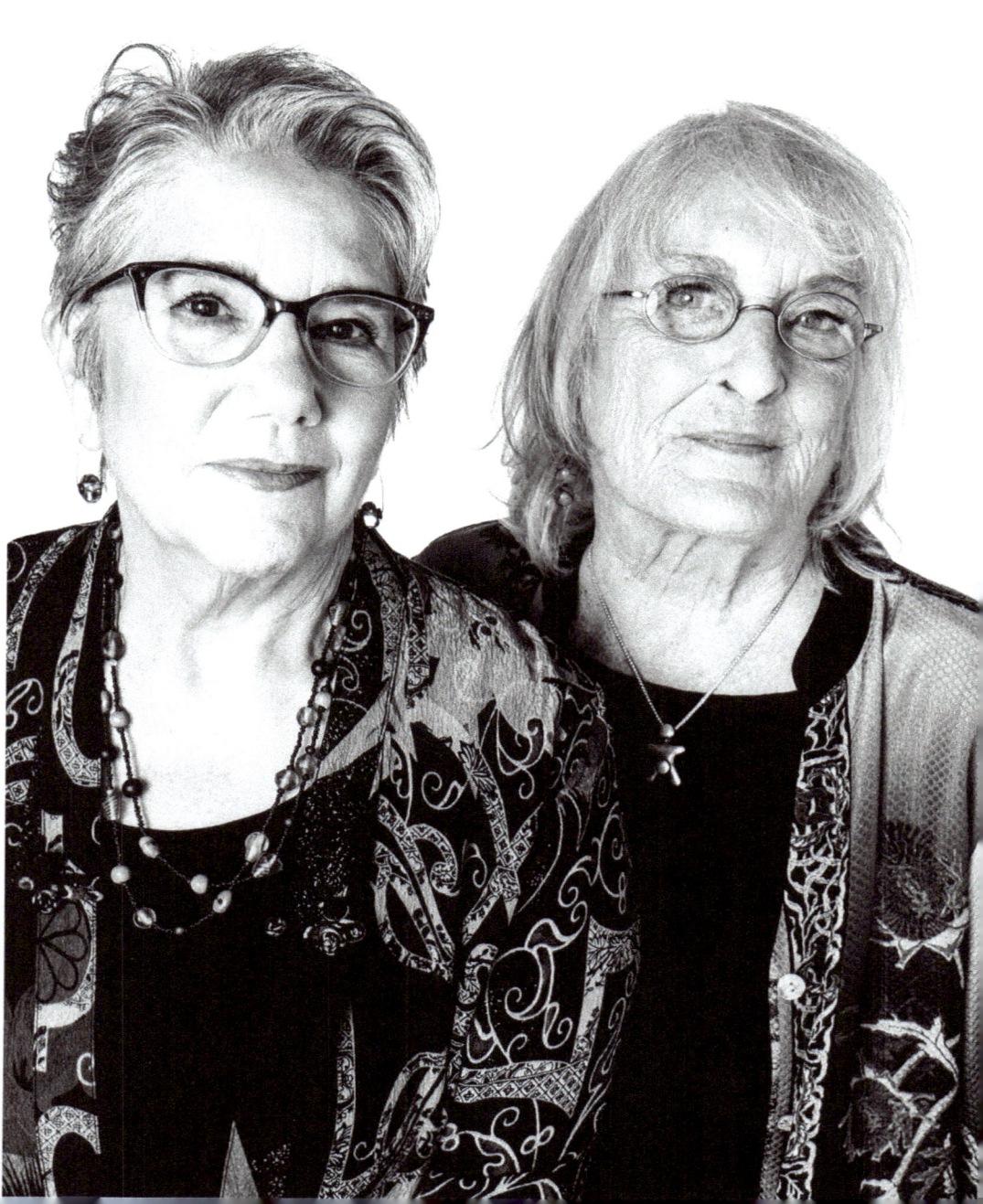

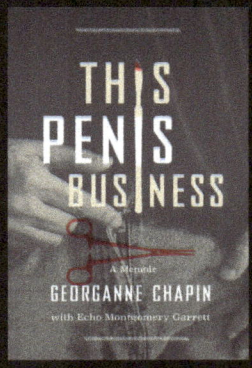

"I wrote the book to answer a question my friend Lucie Saunders asked me nearly two decades ago, as I was becoming active in the movement opposing routine medical circumcision of baby boys. Lucie was a neighbor and a retired anthropologist. We became friends and spent a great deal of time together talking about culture, customs, and people. One day not too long before her death in 2008, Lucie asked me, "How did you get into this… *this penis business?*"

"Since then, while leading Intact America, I thought a lot about Lucie's question. What seemed obvious to me—it makes no sense to routinely amputate a normal body part from a baby boy—didn't seem to occur to most other Americans I knew. Nor did most Americans know that the United States is the only country in the 'developed' world where doctors carry out this surgery routinely. And so, I felt compelled to explore the reasons I'd gotten into "this penis business.'"
—**Georganne Chapin, Founding Executive Director of Intact America**

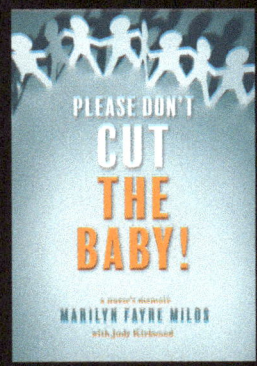

When **Marilyn Fayre Milos**, then an obstetrical nursing student and mother of three circumcised sons, witnessed a circumcision in 1979 she was shocked.

"The doctor looked into my eyes and said, **'There is no medical reason for doing this.'**….Having been awakened to the unnecessary trauma of circumcision, would I simply be a witness to something I knew deep in my soul was a travesty and injustice to a tiny baby delivered into our care and protection? Impossible! I had to do something about it! This was my life-changing moment."
—**Marilyn Fayre Milos,** *Please Don't Cut the Baby! A Nurse's Memoir*

Pressure FROM CULTURE IS INTENSE.

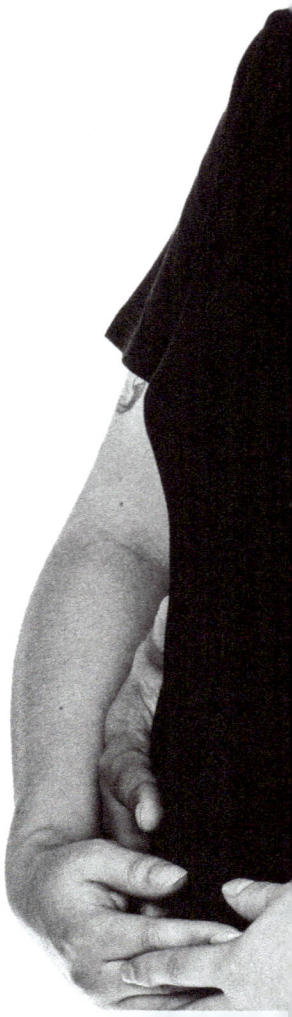

When an expectant parent in the U.S. hears the words: **"You are having a boy,"** the solicitations from medical professionals to consent to circumcision, this "routine procedure" soon follow. An IA Qualtrics survey showed that a pregnant woman is solicited 8 times before her baby boy is born to agree to this irreversible surgery, which is classified as cosmetic and has no medical benefit.

For Black and Latina expectant mothers, the rate of solicitation is even higher.

Male genital cutting of infants and children under the age of consent is a violation of children's rights and perpetuated by the pursuit of profits.

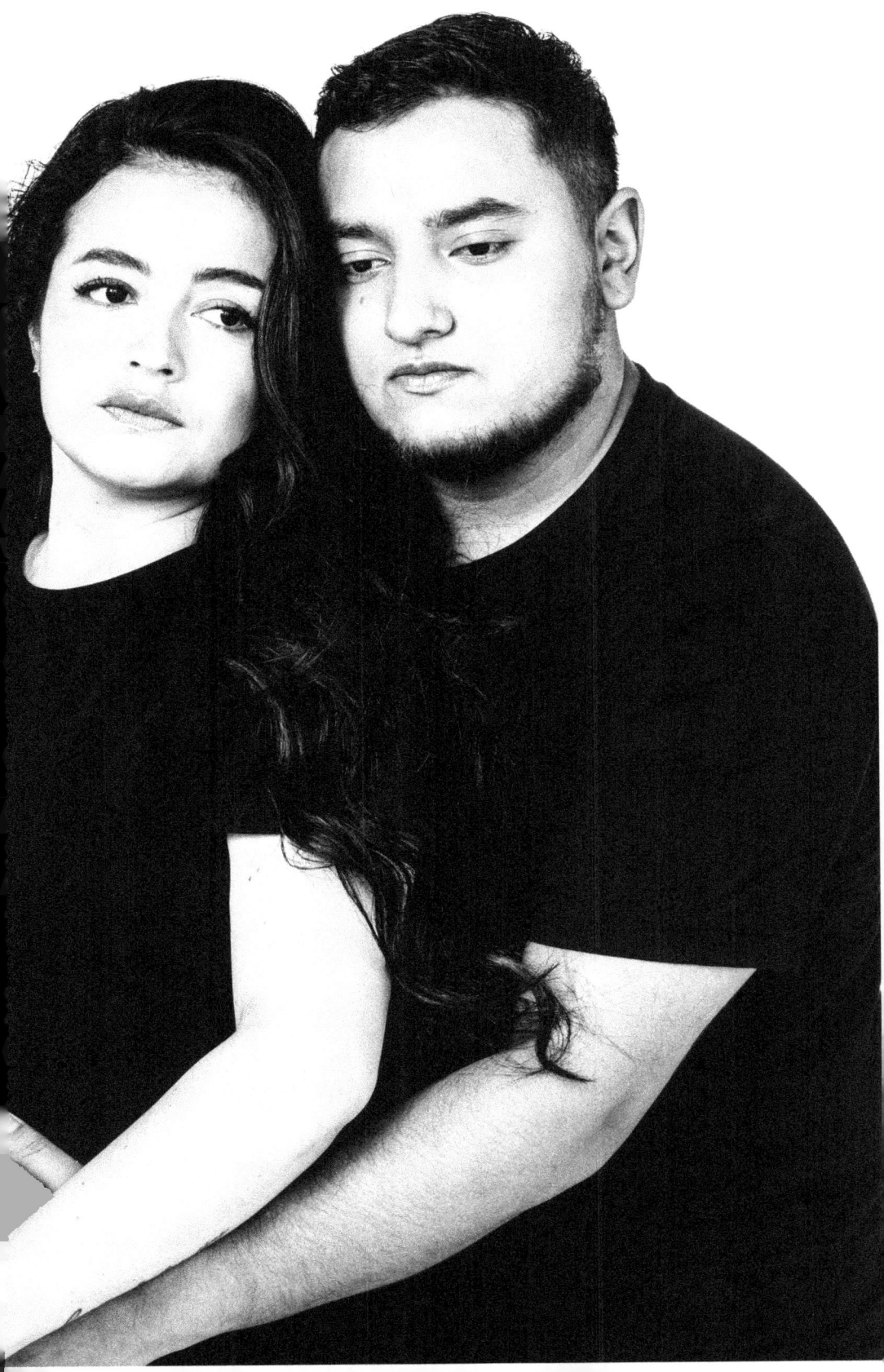

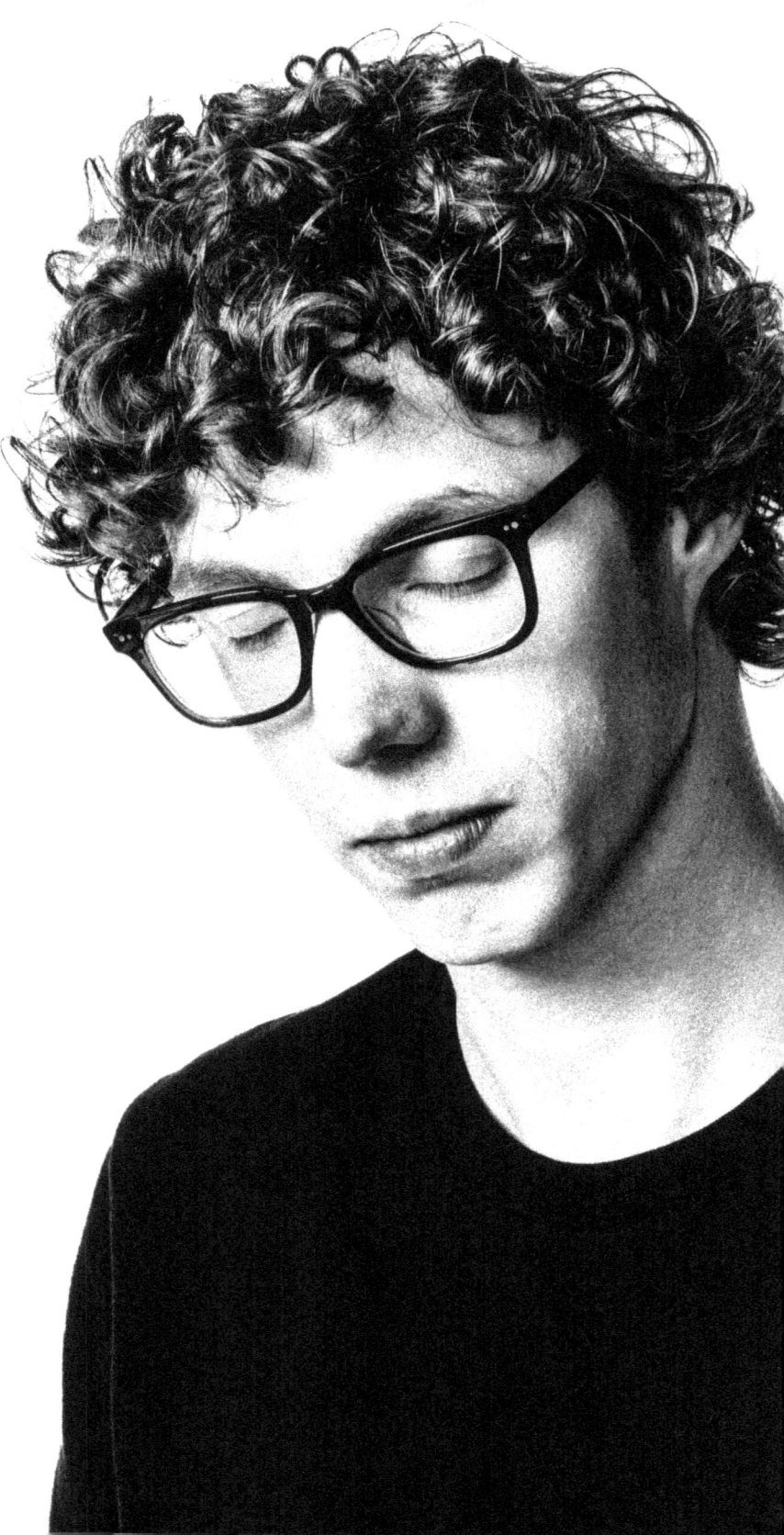

Pressure COMES FROM FAMILY MEMBERS.

Men want their sons to "look like" them. Because circumcision is so deeply embedded in our culture in the US, many people have never seen an intact penis with its foreskin, the natural protective covering for the glans. In fact, many medical books in the U.S. fail to show male genitalia with an intact foreskin.

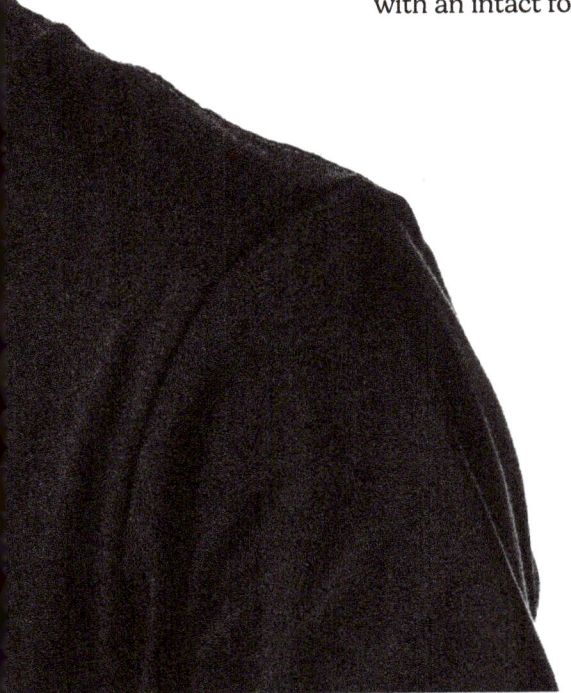

Pressure
COMES FROM PEERS AND SEXUAL PARTNERS.

Young men who are intact are often bullied for "looking different." We've heard a wide range of stories from the under-30 crowd on this topic.

Kishan Patel, a successful entrepreneur who immigrated from India at the age of three months, was seriously investigating circumcision when he met Kelly Floyd, who had become an intactivist at age 18 and is now IA's community programs manager. "If I had not met Kelly when I did, I probably would have done it, because I had gotten so much criticism."

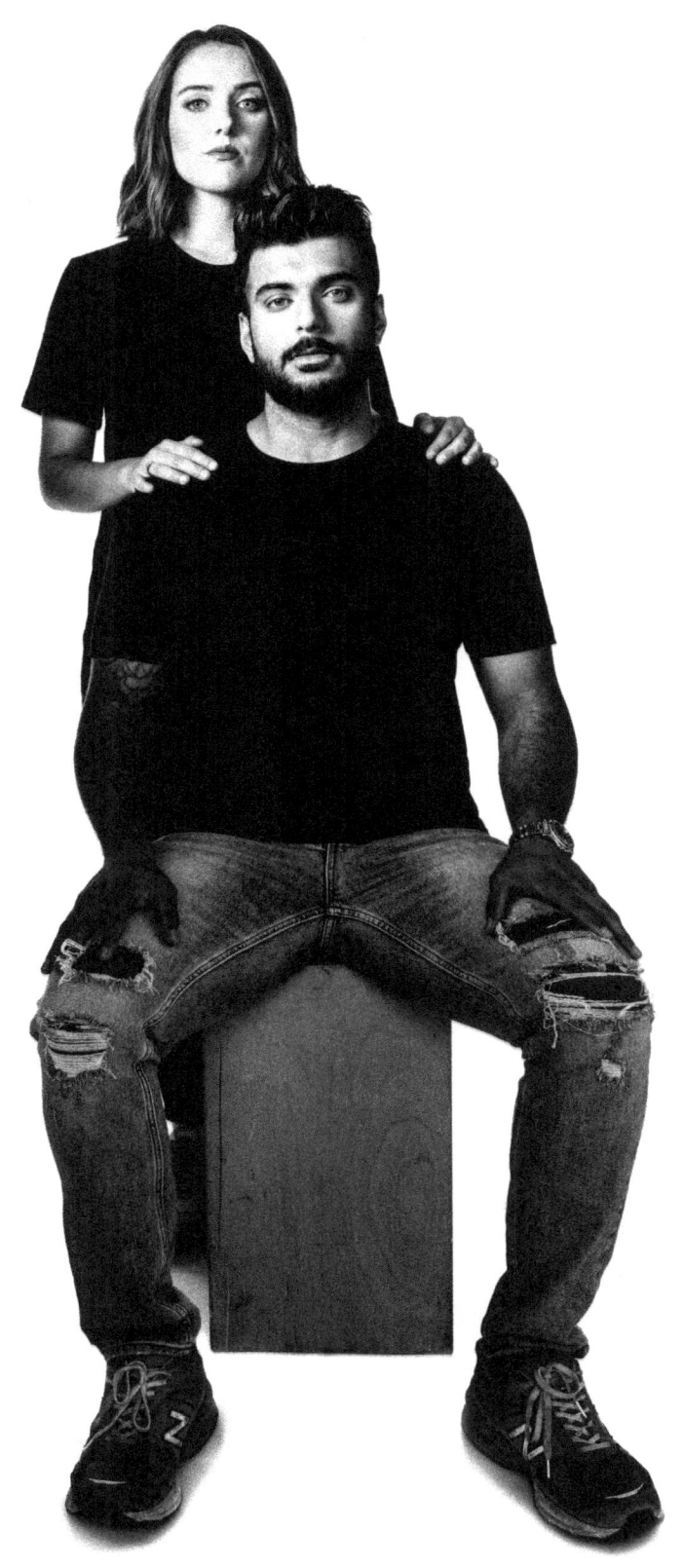

"Let's respect babies' bodies from day one, and not when they finally have a voice, and can say, 'I don't like that.' By then, It's too late. You've already made a life-altering choice for an infant.

When we did our deep dive into circumcision, my husband said, 'I will never do that to my kids. I don't want to risk that.' He and I both feel sad for him as a baby, that it was done to him without his consent and choice. His mother apologized to him when we went down this path with our babies. She said, 'I was wrong, and I made a bad choice for you, and I'm sorry.' My three teenage sons are very vocal about being left whole and thank us for it."
—Angela Orenczak

Angela Orenczak holds a circumstraint, used to immobilize the baby during the surgery.

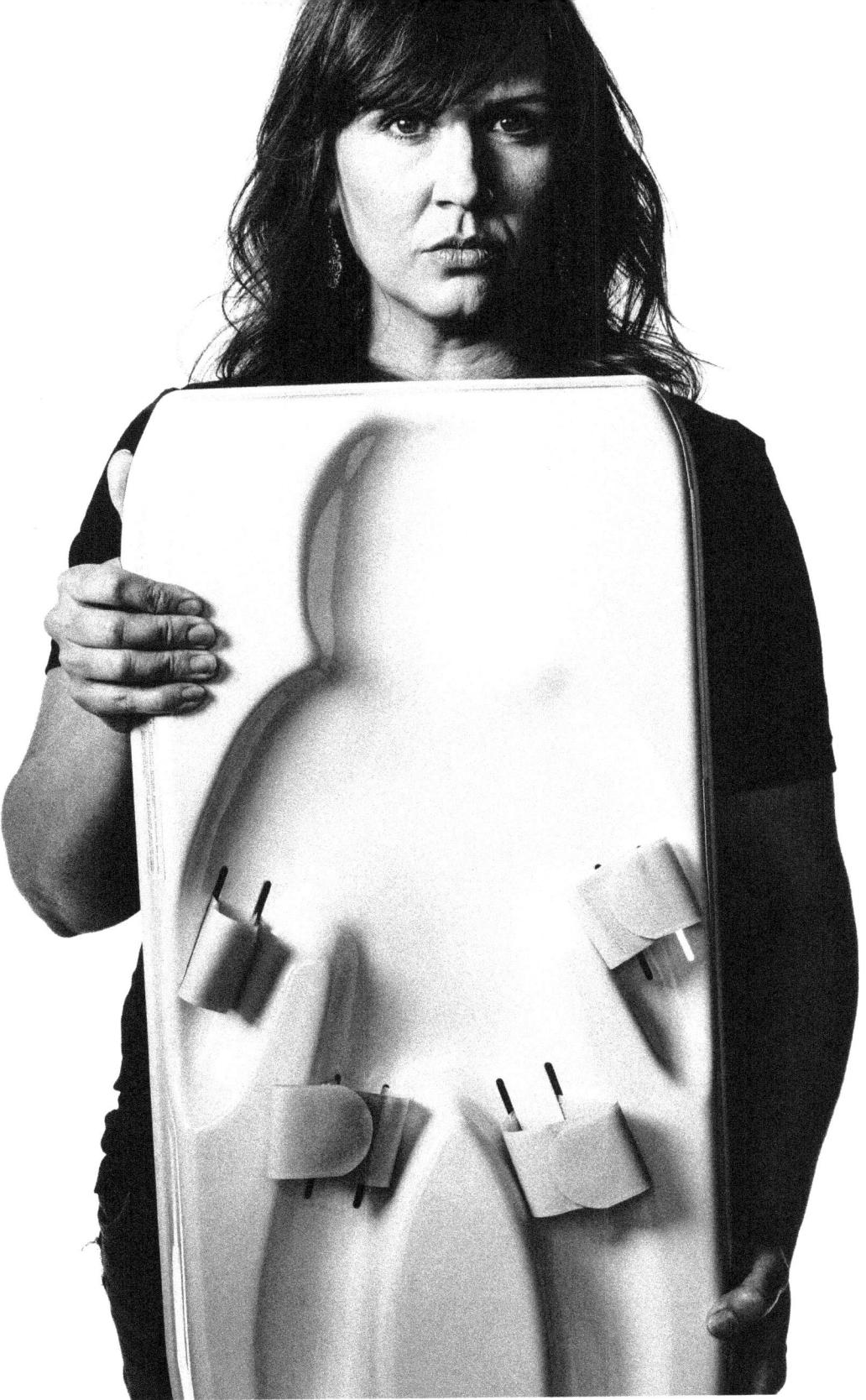

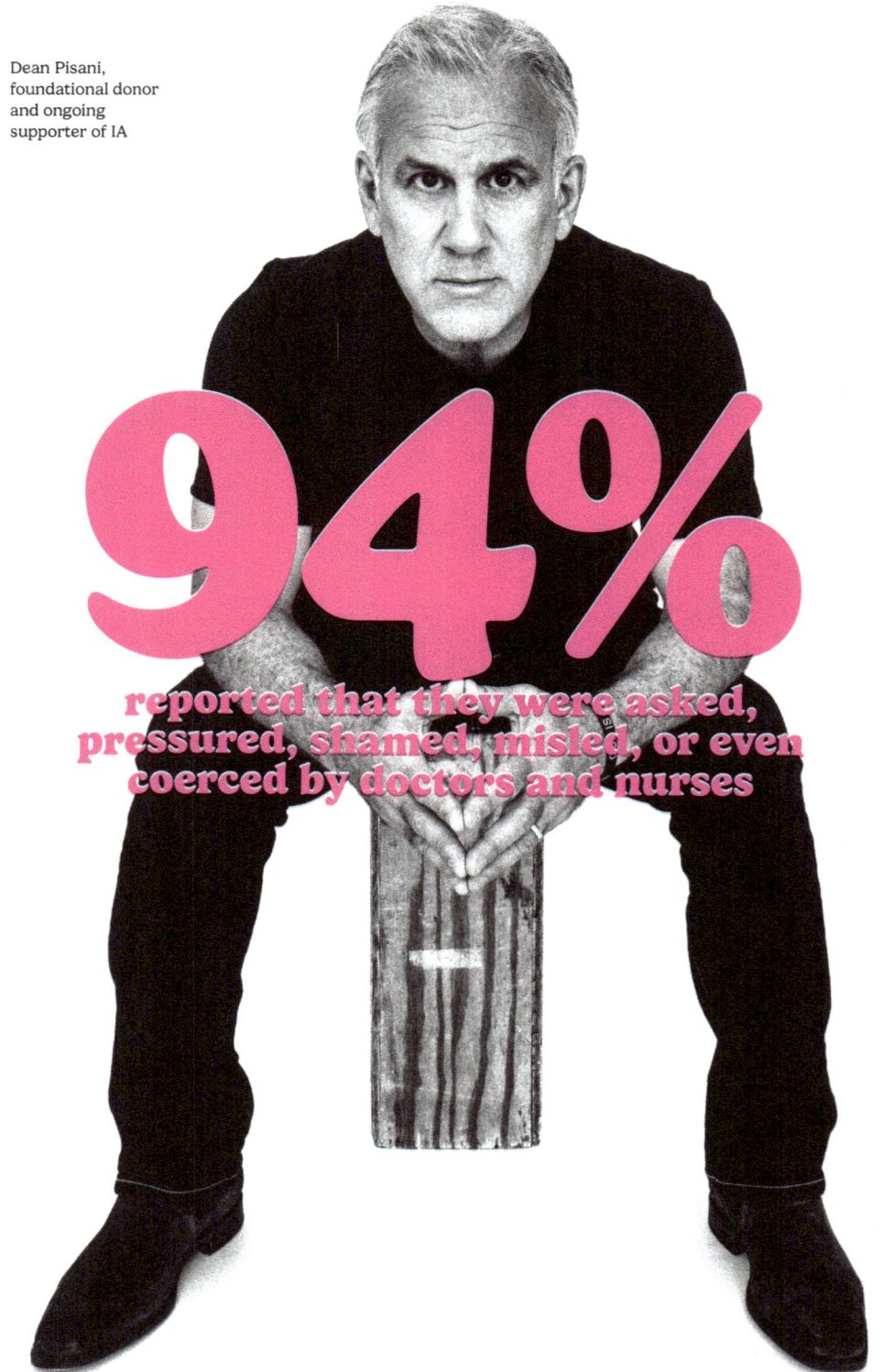

Dean Pisani, foundational donor and ongoing supporter of IA

94% reported that they were asked, pressured, shamed, misled, or even coerced by doctors and nurses

WHY WOULD WE DO THAT?

In IA's 2020 survey of a national, random sample of 2,519 women, who'd given birth to boys between 2017 and 2020, **94 percent** reported that they were **asked, pressured, shamed, misled, or even coerced by doctors and nurses** in healthcare settings to "consent" to circumcision.

When their Ob/Gyn casually said, "If it's a boy, you're going to circumcise, right?" to Dean Pisani and his wife Jackie, a nurse at the time, the couple looked at each other puzzled.

"Why would we do that?" asked Dean.

The doctor shrugged and said, "Everybody does it."

"That's not a good reason," said Dean. "The answer is no."

Dean found a calling. He frequently made donations to Marilyn Fayre Milos' **National Organization of Circumcision Information Resource Centers (NOCIRC)** and eventually spearheaded the talks that led to the formation of **Intact America** and became our foundational donor.

Imagine if more parents saw the tools and circumstraint that are used during this *painful* unnecessary surgery.

Tools of the infant circumcision trade

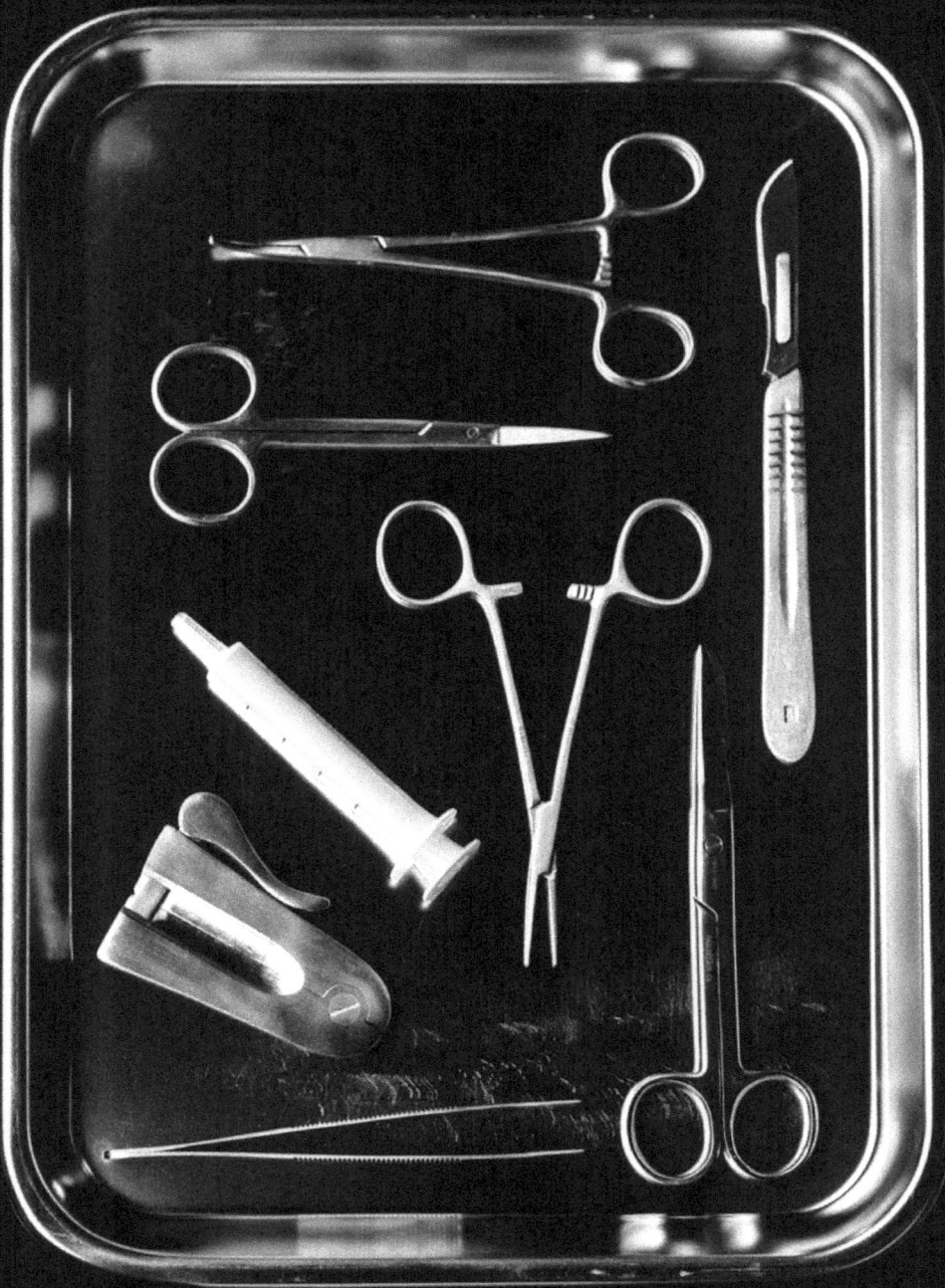

If you are an intact minority, you are a minority

x2

For Eduardo Cardoso, a U.S. Marine and actor, the bullying started in middle school where he was one of the only Latinos and was intact. "I was insecure and even thought about getting circumcised, but I had a close friend, whose mom was Mexican, too, and she talked to me about it. God made me this way and that's enough."

"I've heard teenage girls say hateful things about boys who are not circumcised, and seen educated professional women, including mothers of sons, grimace in disgust at the mention of an intact penis."
—Georganne Chapin in *This Penis Business*

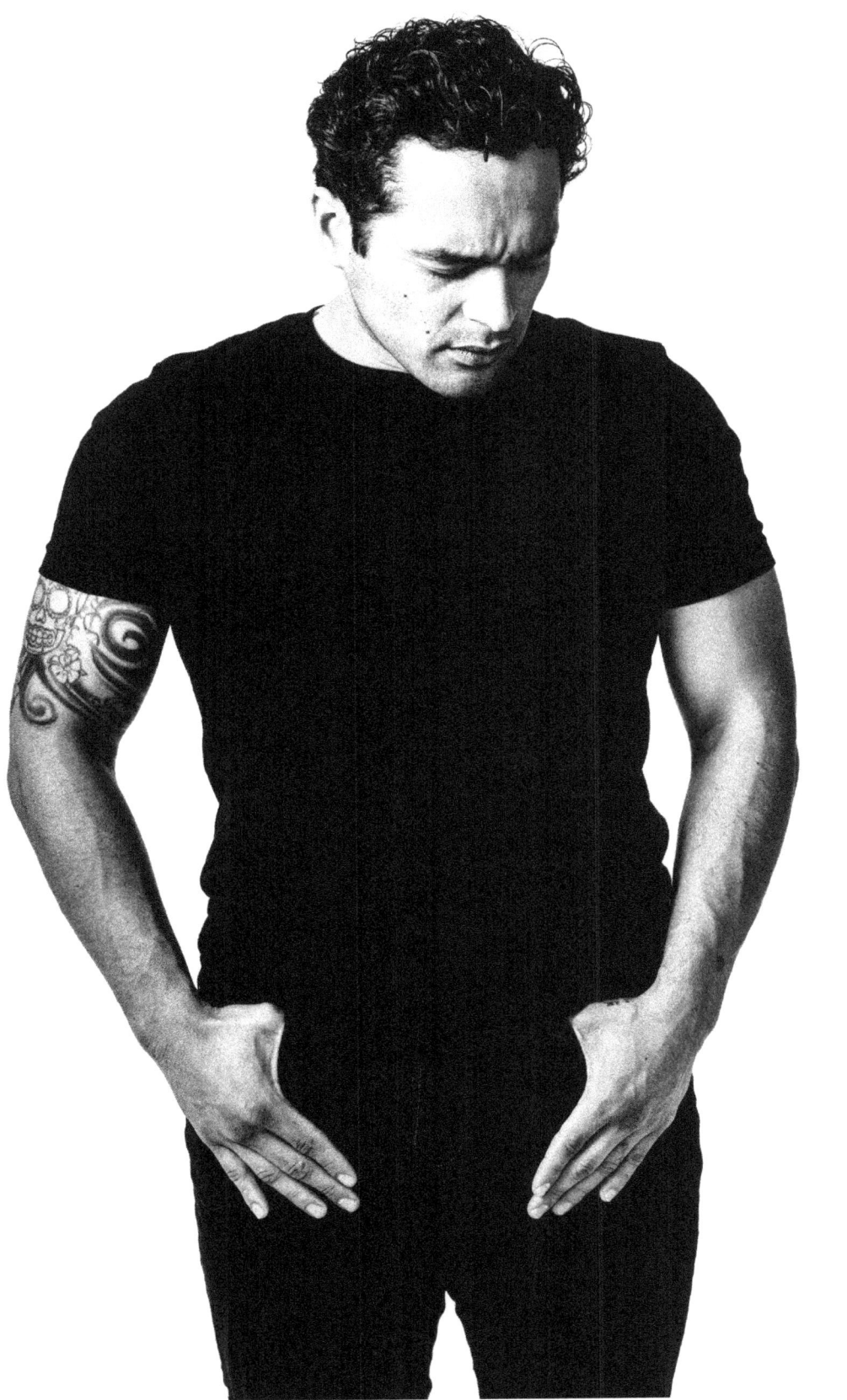

SO JUST HOW BIG IS THIS PENIS BUSINESS?
HUGE.

Board member Dan Bollinger calculated the cost of the circumcision, including doctors' fees, facility bills, and more, and then added: the cost of circumcision repairs (called "revisions by the industry); erectile dysfunction drugs (circumcised men are 4.5 times more likely to be diagnosed with erectile dysfunction; and personal lubricants (a circumcised penis is drier than an intact penis). **Considering that approximately 1.4 million baby boys' foreskins are amputated each year**, Bollinger estimated that total money spent in 2020 as a direct result of circumcision was

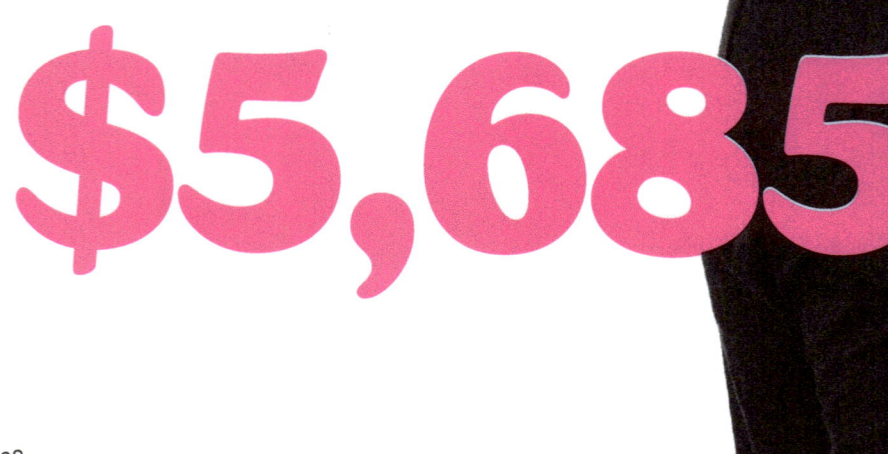

$5,685,

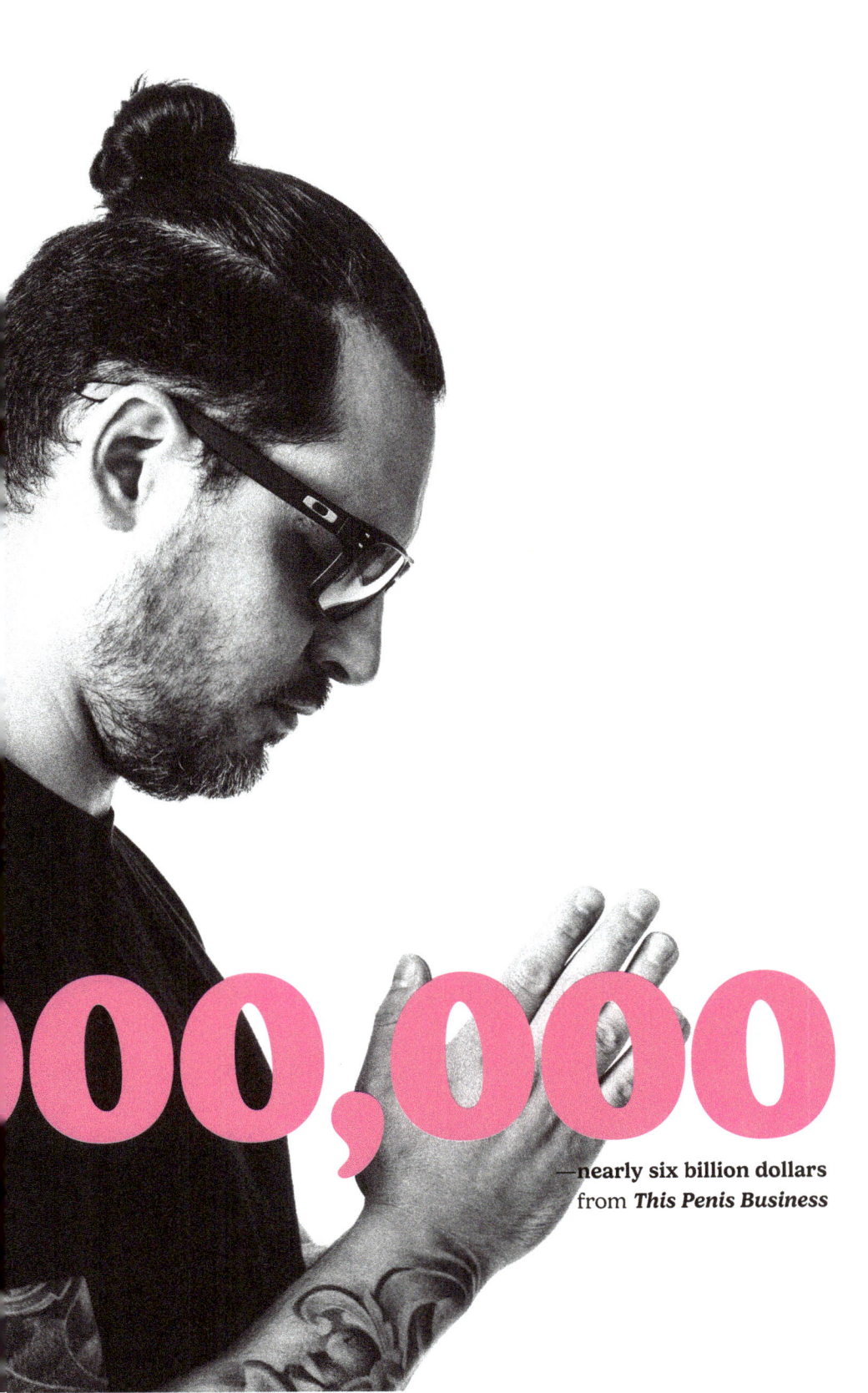

00,000

—nearly six billion dollars
from *This Penis Business*

INJURIES CAUSED BY THOSE SWORN TO DO NO HARM

What if those whose sons were injured or maimed for life or those who chose to keep their sons intact found their wishes ignored and their sons' foreskins forcibly retracted had a place to report medical professionals and facilities that were responsible?

We are launching one of our most important undertakings yet: **DoNoHarm.Report,** a public-facing online portal will collect medical malpractice reports related to circumcision solicitation, circumcision injuries, and forcible foreskin retraction.

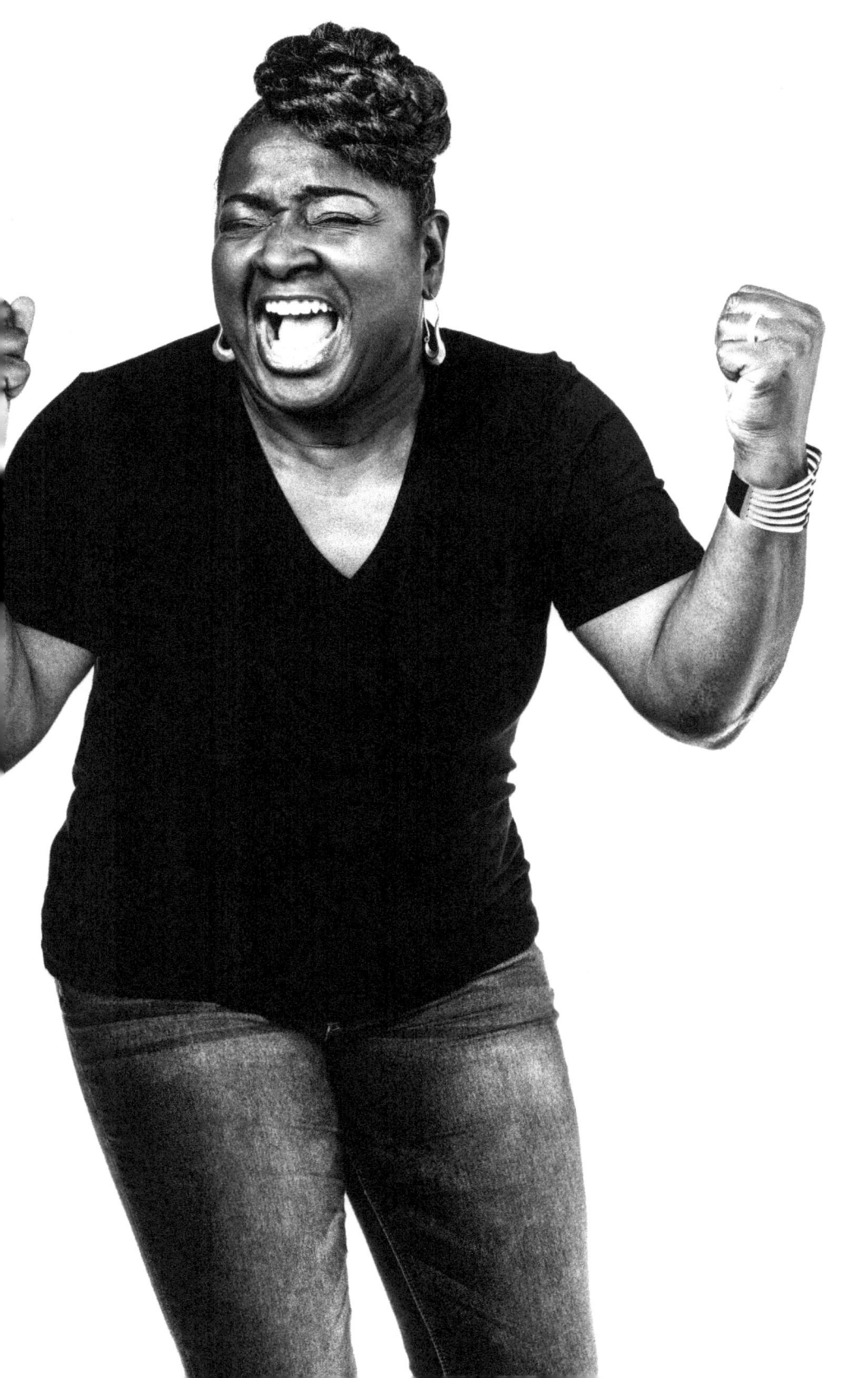

"The doctor who pulled the foreskin down put my son in a lot of pain. His excuse was that it was dirty and needed to be cleaned."

—DoNoHarm.report, surveyed parent

To plan for DoNoHarm's launch, we surveyed parents about how medical providers have treated their intact boys.

DoNoHarm will have the capacity to capture thousands — if not tens of thousands — of these incidents. It will also track complaint responses and non-responses from hospitals, providers, and state regulatory agencies. Then, IA will bring this evidence of medical negligence and abuse to the public's attention — and tear down the American Circumcision Machine from within.

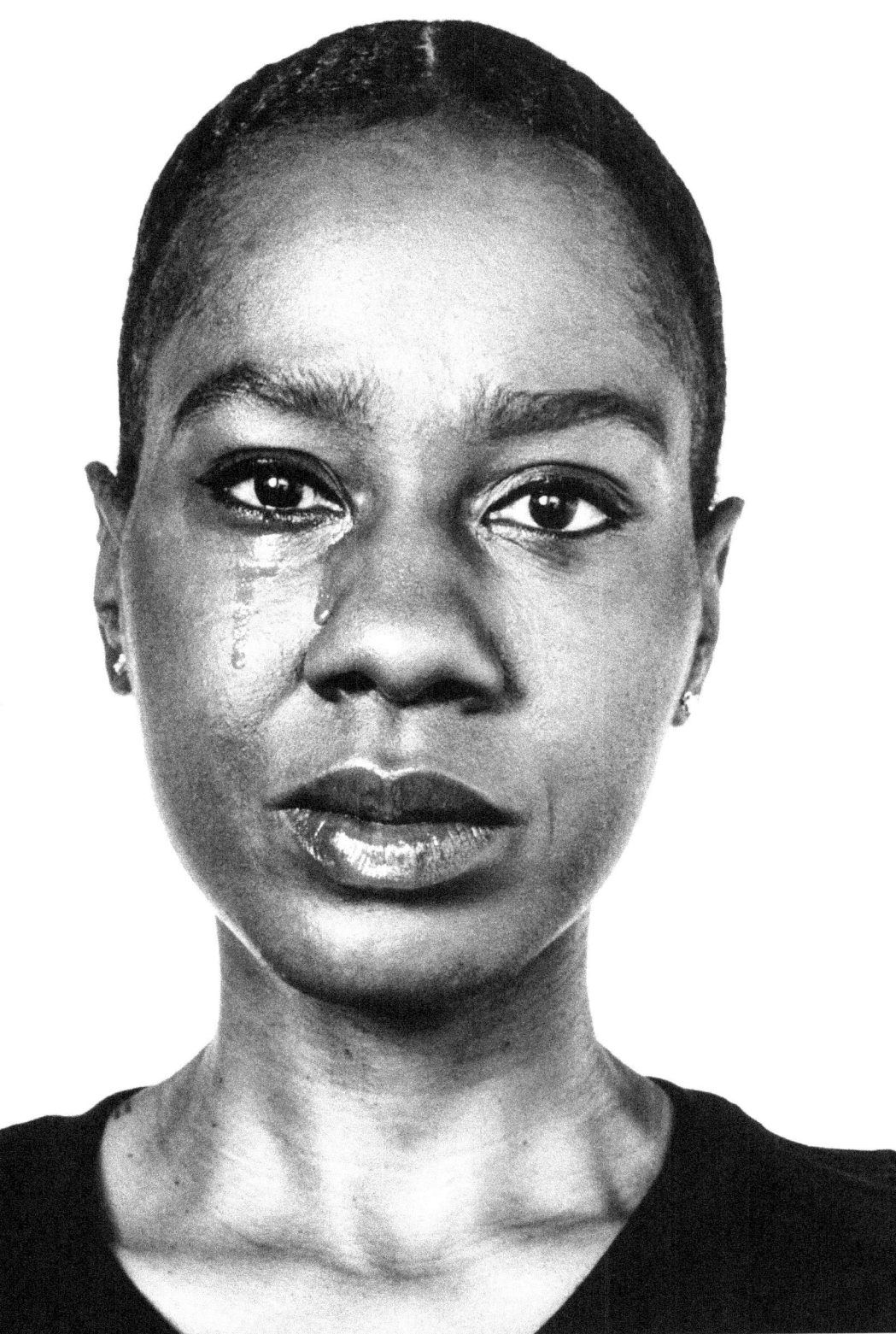

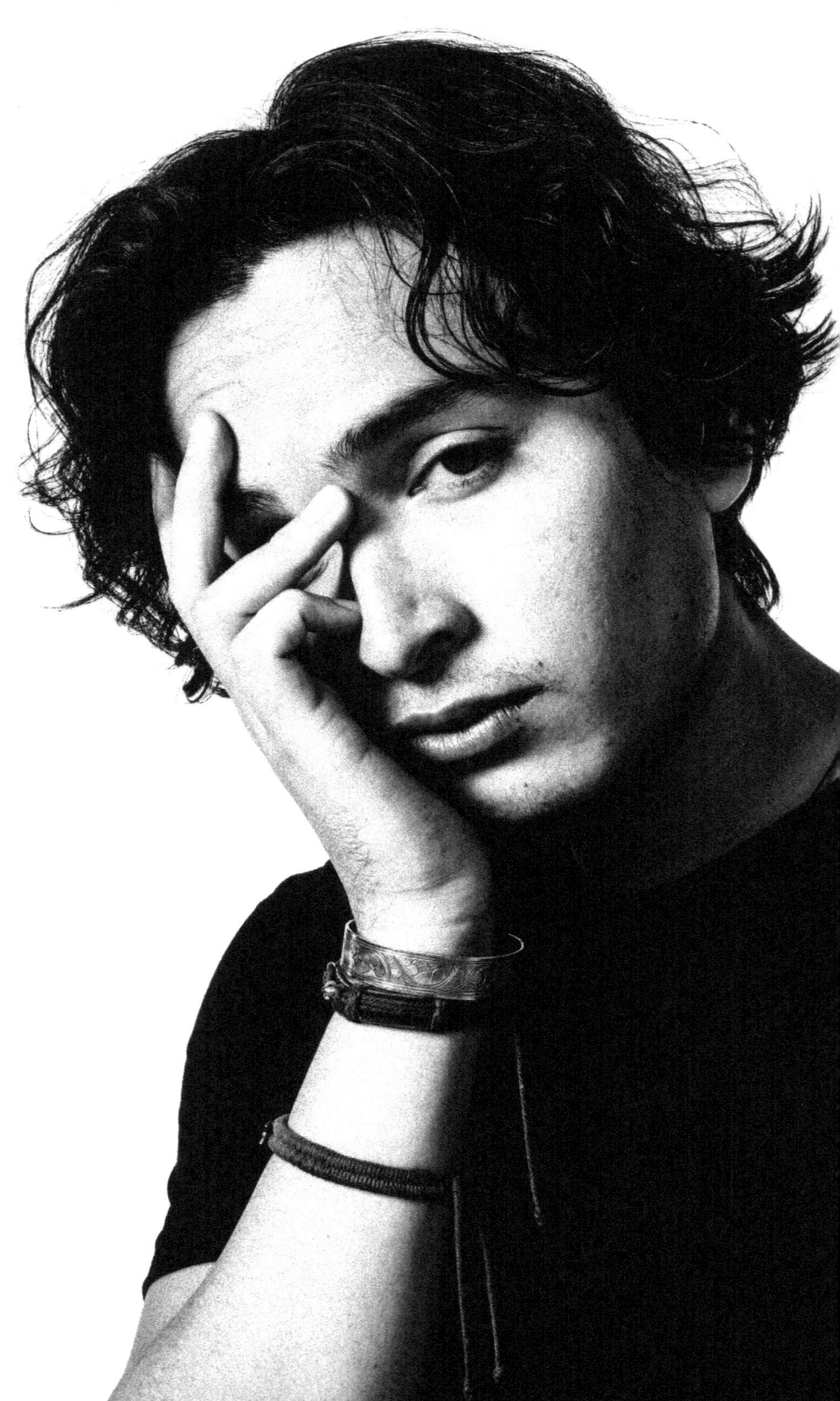

"The whole point of being happy is being happy with oneself and I didn't have the opportunity to be happy with myself because it was taken from me before I could even consent."

There is no time or age limit on those who want to share their stories. We understand that it often takes victims years to process and come forward with what happened.

What if mothers knew that **trauma** from circumcision may have been the root of why they couldn't breastfeed their sons?

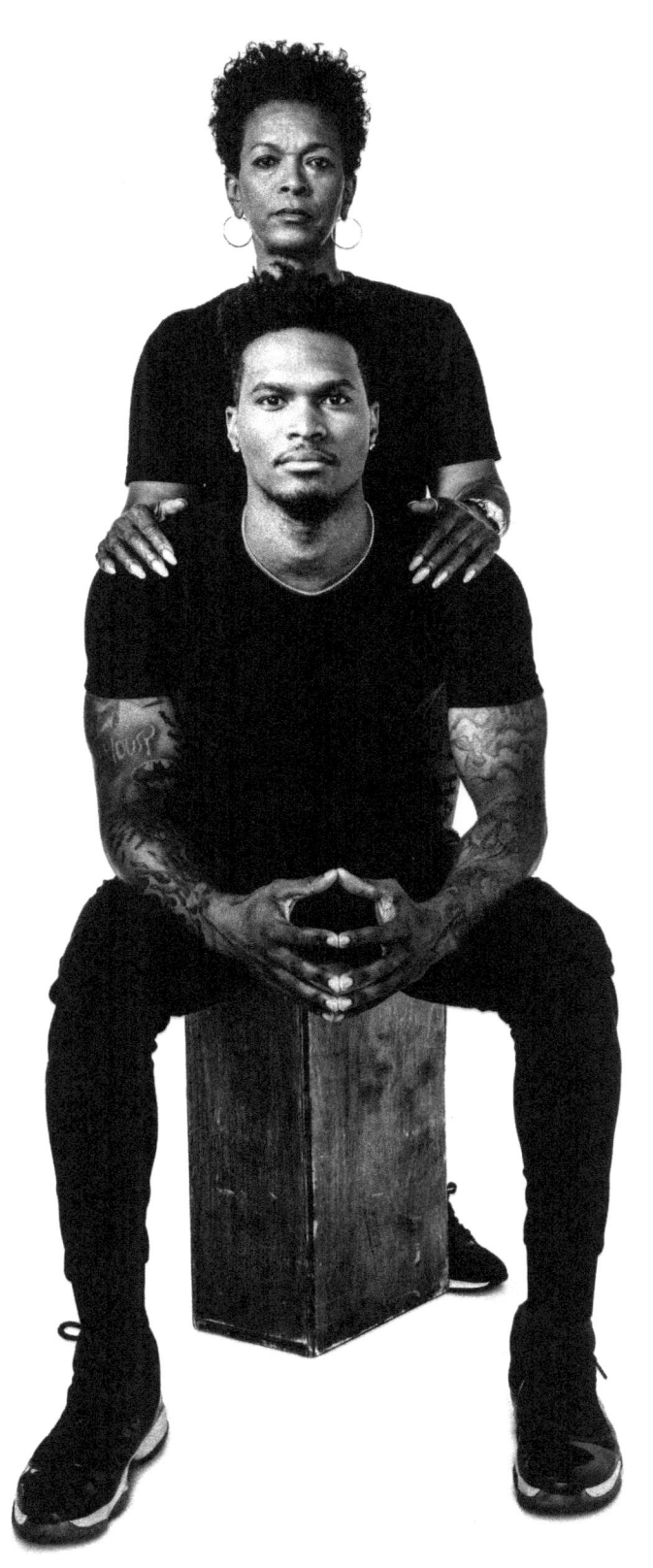

HOW TO MAKE CHANGE.

We've learned over many years that there are so many different angles to the circumcision problem, yet most suffer in silence. What has become obvious is the need for trauma-informed counselors and psychologists who are equipped to address the wounds and scars caused by this assault. Intact America has begun to build a network of mental health professionals who can be a resource for our community.

Together, we can reach the tipping point where removing a boy's foreskin will no longer be the norm.

IntactAmerica.org
To donate, go to IntactAmerica.org/donate

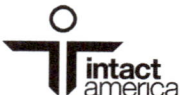

Intact America is a not-for-profit organization registered under Section 501(c)(3) of the Internal Revenue Code. Donations are tax-deductible to the full extent of the law.

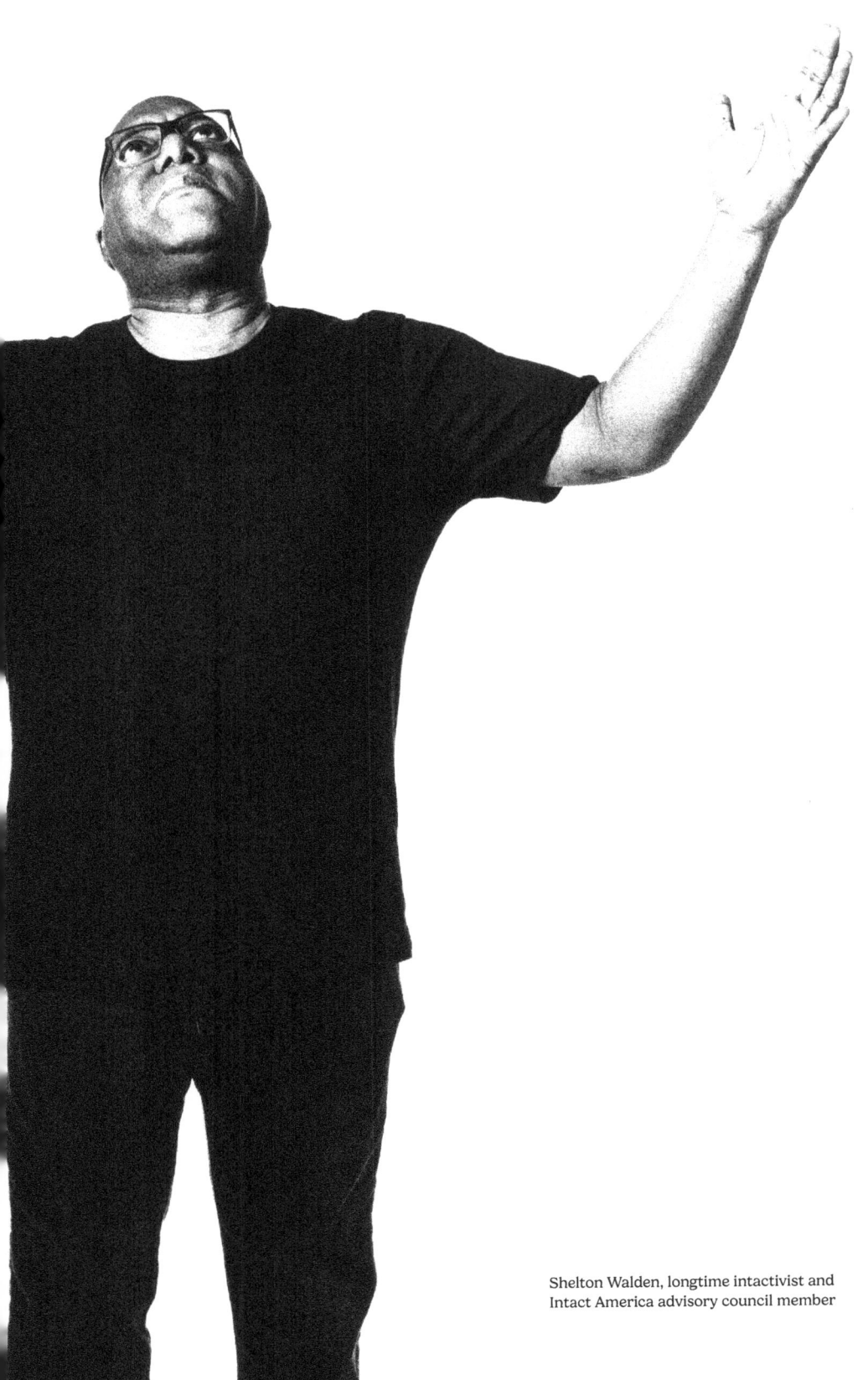

Shelton Walden, longtime intactivist and Intact America advisory council member

SKIN IN THE GAME
CIRCUMCISION CUTS THROUGH US ALL

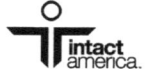

www.ingramcontent.com/pod-product-compliance
Lightning Source LLC
Chambersburg PA
CBHW061811070526
44586CB00024B/2802